T0132409

EYE IQ

303 TIPS FOR EYE HEALTH

REVATHI G. RØNNING

iUniverse, Inc.
New York   Bloomington

EYE IQ
303 tips for eye health

iUniverse books may be ordered through booksellers or by contacting:

iUniverse
1663 Liberty Drive
Bloomington, IN 47403
www.iuniverse.com
1-800-Authors (1-800-288-4677)

Because of the dynamic nature of the Internet, any Web addresses or links contained in this book may have changed since publication and may no longer be valid.

ISBN: 978-1-4401-4554-4 (sc)
ISBN: 978-1-4401-4555-1 (ebk)

Printed in the United States of America

iUniverse rev. date: 12/08/2009

TO MY PARENTS

I am grateful for…
Oh, where do I start?
How can I cover the vast subject?
Let me just say
Thank you with all my heart.

Prevention, Precaution, and Preparation

+

A few simple food and nutrition guidelines

+

Moderate exercise

+

Adequate rest and sleep

=

Good eye health

+

Youthful vitality and vigor

FOREWORD

This book is an attempt at giving simple advice on how to take care of one's eyes. Doctors and hospitals are needed when one is ill but should be avoided when one is well.

If one is healthy and well, it is because of chance. If, on the contrary, one is ill, it is also by chance. Definitely, one can improve the quality of life by observing some simple guidelines.

I understand Ms. Revathi is making an attempt to create awareness of eye care. I have known her for the past twelve years. I have noticed in her the keenness and curiosity to know and to learn. This small book is very much relevant today, as modern medicine has become prohibitively expensive these days. I am sure one who goes through the pages of this small book will find it extremely interesting.

I congratulate Ms. Revathi and wish her all success.

Dr. S. Madhusudanan, MD
Former Professor of Medicine
Medical College and Hospitals
Thiruvananthapuram-695011
Kerala
India

PREFACE

My best friend went to an eye institute when she was eight. She used to wear thick glasses. I think she was the only one in the whole school that sported such thick glasses. The thick glasses were replaced by ordinary glasses when she returned after two months. We spent many hours discussing this. Even at eight, I was a firm believer in prevention (thank you, Mom and Dad, for instilling this in me), and I wanted details. She described one of the exercises (Eyexercise 1) in detail. I took notes. I wanted to be a writer, and I knew I'd use it someday.

During my teens, I filled a few notebooks full of health tips—most of them from real-life observations and first hand experiences. The first one—tips for healthy eyes—grew bigger and bigger. When I was fifteen, one of my neighbors went to an institute and came back sans spectacles. I spent time with him too.

One of my neighbors was absent-minded and had to change his glasses quite often. I saw him neglect caring for his glasses so often that I began to advise him. The tips for glasses are from the eighties.

I grew up in a hot and humid area. Unlike colder countries, it was quite common to get minor eye problems during the summer months. Most of the remedies are from that time.

My friend's illiterate grandmother could see that I had a fever by just looking at my bright shiny eyes. Jaundice (and many other liver disorders) brings about a yellow tinge to the eyes. The doctors in India always pulled the lower eyelid down to check for anemia. The eye is a vital organ that reflects health. It also reflects mental health. By observing the eyes of a child, one can learn if he or she has good mental health.

At sixteen, I voluntarily took a weeklong first aid course, which was mandatory for the science students. Not only did I ace both theory and practicals, but I also managed to impress all the guest lecturers (mostly surgeons from the main hospital). Everyone was disappointed that I did not choose the medical field. Even then, I firmly believed that health and fitness was not just the absence of disease. It was much more than just conventional medicine. The eye surgeon was very impressed. He agreed to give me an informal interview. More than a third of the tips in this book were discussed and approved by him. He found it strange that I was going from the angle of prevention rather than cure. Then, I finished school and forgot all about the notebook.

In the university, my roommate borrowed a pair of colored contact lenses and got an infection. She thought it was OK, as the owner did not have any infections. After all, it was just for one evening. She recovered within a week, but this incident made me restart my eye health observations.

After university, I began to work in Delhi. Unlike my native place, here the temperature could rise to 43 or 45 degrees Celsius during summers. When the temperature rose to 40 degrees Celsius, I was consuming cucumber every day. I was dispersing advice and cucumber slices to happy recipients. I had been told by my mother and grandmother that cucumber was good during summers. My cousins told me it was a vegetable for beautiful skin. During summers we did eat a lot of cucumbers.

Prevention is often a family trait. One of my neighbors had two small children. The parents were not too keen on prevention techniques. I tried to warn them that they should be careful and also teach their children eye safety. Some of my tips about safety are from that period. Unfortunately, they did not listen to me. They had multiple emergency visits one year. During one such visit, the surgeon who stitched up the wound managed to scare them. He warned them about the worst-case scenarios. I was happy to see that they finally began to inculcate prevention into their daily life.

I began to use the computer and got more tips. When I taught computer courses, I was concerned with ergonomics—especially when I saw twenty bad-postured students in front of me.

The connection between diet, lifestyle, and eye health is yet to be documented—at least in the scientific world. Many of the sceptics out there might not be willing to change their diet or lifestyle until it's too late. Quite a few experiments have been and are being conducted. Hopefully in a few years, we'll take good care of ourselves. We might even care for our bodies with the similar respect we have for our cars and houses.

Thank you for buying this book. This is a labor of love. I hope this book will prevent incidents and will contribute to better eye health. Eye health and vision are vital antiageing techniques. I firmly believe in the quality of life, however long it may be.

This book is far from complete. But I hope that it's a start to your optimal eye health.

INTRODUCTION

The eye is the jewel of the body.

~ Henry David Thoreau

Overused, overworked, and underappreciated ... I can go on. No, it's not a documentary. It's the story of our eyes. Our eyes are among our most precious possessions. We search for miracles high and low. We don't realize that each time we see something, it's a miracle in itself.

I was waiting for my father. His cataract was being removed. I was too tense to read and did not want to pace up and down. Instead I began to observe the people passing by and the others in that packed room. Most of them either squeezed their eyes, or yanked off the crusts, or touched their eyes. One mom helped her toddler son to take off his crust, and he began to howl. They were waiting to see the eye surgeon. One guy went to the vending machine and bought his diabetic mother a sweet soda. I overheard their conversation—that's how I know this—and she thought it was OK. After all, she was good with her diet. The water cooler there was broken. Except for the toddler's mom and me, none of the people carried water bottles. Some of them had to wait for a couple of hours, at least. Of course, they could always get a sugary soda when they got very thirsty.

OK, they were not enlightened. What about the hospital workers? Sorry to say that they too did not take simple preventive steps. One of the eye doctors (maybe he was a newbie?) opened the door to look for a patient, when he got the urge to scratch and squeeze his left eye. For convenience, he let go of the knob, switched hands, and then scratched his eye with the same hand that had just held the doorknob. The chrome did not look filthy, but it had been touched by many persons within the past hour.

Most people want the best for themselves and those they care about. Education does not enlighten us how to take care of our eyes. Even those in the medical field, those who know how to solve problems when they occur, are not enlightened about the prevention issues that can prevent or at least delay and reduce problems.

Do my experience and knowledge and real-life happenings support this book? Yes. Am I an authority in this field? No. Why did I write this book? I know that many people can benefit from these tips. I want to instill the concept of prevention, and I believe that this book will go a long way in doing so. I believe that this book is thought-provoking and will make a very good gift. Does this book take the place of medical advice? No, definitely not. But you are welcome to discuss this with your doctor so you may improve your eye health.

I have my bachelor's in psychology and have done a basic medicine course: anatomy and physiology. I have also done a food and nutrition diploma course. In addition to these, I also hold a Microsoft Office User Specialist Certification. I am a qualified Medical Secretary. I have taught Microsoft Office programs and have also worked as a PA to the ambassador in Foreign Service. I also offer coaching sessions and nutritional consultant services. The spectrum is broad. I have worked with diplomats, engineers, educators, medical professionals, etc. One common factor is that very few people are aware of eye health. Some are aware of good nutrition, while some others take a few precautions, but most are ignorant about many preventive factors.

Eyes seem to be a low item on our priority list. We have procured more daylight hours with the invention of the electric bulb, more strain on the eye with the TV, Internet, etc. To make it worse, we've reduced our sleep hours and also reduced our manual exertions. I do love my computer and am happy that the washing machine was invented. But if these devices could make life simpler, shouldn't we lounge about more and sleep more and relax our eyes more? We do none of these. Instead, we cram more activities into our waking hours (which have been increased) and strain our eyes even more.

Eye surgeons are busy people. Though they want the best for you, they barely have time to check your eyes and find solutions. Somewhere along the line, prevention has been firmly tossed out. They are not alone. Very few doctors have the time to talk about prevention to patients. If something can be fixed, they step up and fix it. We need a few prods toward prevention. I hope this book is one such reminder.

Cataract surgery has become such an everyday phenomenon that we fail to appreciate the miracle. I am thrilled that this procedure is possible at all. It may not be possible to prevent all cataracts. But some, if not most, of the incidents of cataracts can be prevented. I hope each of you who pick up this book discusses this with your friends and family. If you're a parent, teach your children good eye habits.

If you're an adult, help your parents cultivate some good eye habits. This may reduce multiple visits to the surgery. Though most of the eye problems are fixable these days, prevention still is better than cure.

I firmly believe that quality of life is very important. It is vital that you live a wonderful life rather than just a long one. Vision is a vital youth factor. Taking care of your eyes is a start. If you want to delay ageing , this book is for you. If you value your health and believe that prevention is the key, then this book is for you. This book is for anybody and everybody who wants to take care of their eyes. Take care of them and they'll serve you well for a lifetime. These tips will help you retain your precious treasures for a youthful old age.

Our eyes are our windows to the world. Most of our knowledge comes through our eyes (in sighted people). When we meet someone, our first impression includes their eyes. Eyes express our emotions and can speak louder than words. Our eyes are our most precious possessions. Let's take care of them.

Please visit me at:

http://www.startlivingtoday.org

You have the gift of vision. Do your best to keep your eyes healthy. Buying this book is a start. Good luck.

The best six doctors anywhere

And no one can deny it

Are **sunshine**, **water**, **rest**, and **air**

Exercise and **diet**.

These six will gladly you attend

If only you are willing

Your mind they'll ease

Your will they'll mend

And charge you not a shilling.

~ *Nursery rhyme quoted by Wayne Fields,* **What the River Knows,** *1990*

> *We are what we repeatedly do. Excellence then, is not an act, but a habit.*
>
> *~ Aristotle*

1. Whenever you can, whenever you remember, just close your eyes for a few seconds. Your overworked eyes will welcome these short breaks. Make this habit yours.

2. Make it a habit not to squeeze your eyes or eyelids on waking up. Pushing sleep out—or is it welcoming wrinkles?

3. The skin around the eyes is extremely delicate—avoid pulling, scratching, and unnecessary touching.

4. Don't tug the hard crust (gunk) that forms at the corner of the eye. Gently splash cool or lukewarm water, if necessary, and remove it with a clean tissue.

5. After showering, pat your eyes dry gently. Avoid rubbing vigorously with your towel.

In a way, staring into a computer screen is like staring into an eclipse. It's brilliant and you don't realize the damage until its too late.

~ Bruce Sterling

6. Don't stare at your computer monitor for many hours. Take a mini break every ten to twelve minutes. Get up and stretch. Close your eyes and take a few deep breaths. Take a break every half hour. Get up; walk for a minute or two; get some water or herbal tea.

7. Try to have one day a week free from the computer. Or just use it minimally.

8. Be ergonomic. The right height for your monitor is vital. If the monitor too high or too low, it can tire the neck, shoulders, back, and the muscles that support your head. This means more eyestrain.

9. The top of the monitor should be at or slightly below eye level. The center of the computer monitor should normally be located 15 to 20 degrees below horizontal eye level.

10. Lighting is very important to minimize eyestrain while using the computer. It is preferable to have soft lighting from above and to the side, not directly behind the monitor or behind you.

11. Avoid glare from windows or other lamps on your monitor. Glare causes eyestrain.

TV will never be a serious competitor for radio because people must sit and keep their eyes glued on a screen; the average American family hasn't time for it.

~ *Anon., from* New York Times, *1939*

12. Do not face windows or bright light sources. You will be unconsciously alternating between bright window light and your monitor. The result will be multiple strains on your eyes.

13. Place the keyboard directly in front of the monitor to avoid eyestrain.

14. Keep your monitor clean. Use a microfiber cloth and avoid chemicals.

15. Spectacles plus many hours of computer use every day is not a good combination. Your doctor may prescribe special glasses.

16. Sitting in front of a computer monitor reduces your blinking rate and causes dry eyes. Every few minutes, turn away from the monitor and consciously blink very slowly.

Lack of activity destroys the good condition of every human being, while movement and methodical physical exercise save it and preserve it.

~ Plato

17. Regular aerobic exercise is vital for the health of your eyes. A brisk forty to forty to fifty minute daily walk will suffice. Start with ten minutes and increase gradually.

18. Regular exercise can help ward off diabetes (type 2), which may lead to eye conditions.

19. Always consult your physician before you start any exercise routine.

*Health is the greatest gift, contentment the greatest
wealth, faithfulness the best relationship.*

~ Buddha

20.   *Eyexercise 1*

Sit comfortably near a window.

Breathe in and out deeply.

Look at the tip of your nose and count slowly to five.

Then look out of the window at something one to two meters (one to two yards) away and count slowly to five.

Then, look at something farther away, say, ten to twenty meters (ten to twenty yards) away.

Then look at the horizon.

Now do this in the reverse order.

Repeat.

> *Everything is for the eye these days: TV, Life, Look, the movies. Nothing is just for the mind. The next generation will have eyeballs as big as cantaloupes and no brain at all.*
>
> **~ Fred Allen**

21. TV: the curse of mankind? It not only makes us couch potatoes and devours our leisure time, but is also a big strain on our eyes.

22. While watching TV, take a break every fifteen minutes. Get up, stretch, and walk for a minute. No movie or serial or documentary, however interesting or well made, is worth more than your eyes.

23. While watching TV, close your eyes for two to three minutes, just counting your deep breaths. Do it every now and then.

24. Get up, walk to another room, and stretch during commercial breaks. How many times do you want to see the same commercial?

25. Adjust the height of your TV. Avoid looking up or down at the TV screen.

26. Place the TV so that it has no glare from other lamps or windows on the screen.

27. Have soft adequate lighting in the TV room. The lighting should not be too bright or behind the TV.

What compels you to stare, night after night, at all the glittering hokum that has been deliberately put together for you?

~ J.B. Priestly

28. Have one TV-free day per week. Whatever reasons you have, you should refuse to switch on the TV that day. Use that evening to relax. Go in for a soak in the tub or listen to your music.

29. Kick some ball with your children. Or visit your parents. Or just relax listening to your favorite music.

30. Take a break from TV. Relax your eyes for an entire week of no TV. Record all the programs you do not want to miss. Use that week to indulge yourself. Take a walk; go rock climbing; read a book; listen to music; get a massage; take a bubble bath; soak your feet; go hiking, mall walking, bowling … the list is endless.

> *Drink to me only with thine eyes,*
> *And I will pledge with mine;*
> *Or leave a kiss but in the cup,*
> *And I'll not look for wine.*
>
> ~ *Benjamin Johnson*

31. Do not apply any cream or oil (other than eye creams) around your eyes. Even face creams can be too harsh for the thin, delicate skin around your eyes.

32. Invest in a good eye cream, preferably an organic cream with minimum (or no) chemicals and no perfume.

33. Apply eye cream after showering and before you put on your makeup.

34. Apply eye cream after removing your makeup. Do it before going to bed.

What is it that you express in your eyes? It seems to me more than all the words I have read in my life.

~ Walt Whitman

35. We have the thinnest skin on our eyelids. Remember this before slathering on makeup.

36. Use eye makeup occasionally—for special occasions. Do not use it on a daily basis if you're not in the entertainment business.

37. Do not borrow or lend eye makeup. If you have to lend an item for an emergency, toss it when it is returned.

38. Replace all eye makeup regularly. If your summer temperature reaches 40 degrees Celsius and you do not store your makeup in the fridge, you ought to throw it out every month. But if you live in a temperate zone or if you store it in the fridge, throw it out every three to four months. Ruthlessly toss them even if they're quite unused.

39. Whenever you open a makeup item, write the date on it. You won't have to tax your memory when you're going through your cabinet.

40. Mascara should be replaced more often, as the wands can harbor bacteria and a scratch on the cornea may lead to a severe infection. Never borrow or lend mascara.

41. Buy only quality eye makeup. Costlier does not always mean better quality.

Good health and good sense are two of life's greatest blessings.

~ *Publilius Syrus*

42.   Read the ingredient list on your eye makeup items. The fewer the chemicals, the better. Again, certain chemicals are bad guys. Read about these chemicals and what they can do to your skin. Make a project out of this and let shopping be an adventure—you are trying to elude these chemicals.

43.   Remove makeup gently before going to bed. Use mild cleansers for this.

44.   If you curl your eyelashes a lot, it can be a good idea to use eyelash oils (applied just like mascara) to feed and repair the eyelashes in between curling treatments.

45.   If you have sensitive skin: Hypo-allergenic cosmetics free of oil, fragrances, or dyes are the best items for eye makeup. Avoid lash-building mascara that lengthen and thicken eyelashes. Avoid oil-based mascara. Use water-based mascara for special occasions.

The eyes have one language everywhere.

~ George Herbert

46. If you use glasses, go to your eye doctor as prescribed.

47. Usually you don't notice that you need an adjustment till it is too late. So, go to your optician every year for a checkup.

48. Use both hands while you put on or take off your glasses, or you might bend one of the hinges.

49. Protect the lenses from being scratched. Always store the glasses in the protective case. Invest in a trendy solid case.

50. Never place the glasses lens side down. In fact, whenever you take off your glasses, put them in the case at once, or use a strap.

51. Wash the glasses in lukewarm soapy water.

52. Use a soft toothbrush to wash the nose pads and handles. Buy a baby toothbrush that is soft and use it exclusively for this.

53. Hairsprays and other sprays can coat the lens on your glasses. Try to remove your glasses to safety while using the sprays.

Happiness is nothing more than good health and a bad memory.

~ Albert Schweitzer

54.   Do you squint when you read or watch TV? Ask your friends or family to observe you.

55.   If you use the computer three or more hours daily, see your doctor about glasses to reduce eyestrain.

56.   If your occupation requires you to have magnification of near objects (plumber, mechanic, etc.), get special glasses.

57.   Special sports glasses can provide protection from injury, and they can improve contrast and enhance vision for sports activities.

Every generation laughs at the old fashions, but follows religiously the new.

~ Henry David Thoreau

58. Always wash your hands with a mild soap or cleanser before your insert or remove your contact lenses. Make sure that your soap has no moisturizer.

59. Insert your lens over a clean towel, so if it drops, you can easily find it and it will still be clean.

60. Clean, rinse, and disinfect your lenses after removal and before wearing them again.

61. Always clean your contact lenses with the recommended sterile solution.

62. Avoid getting tap water on or near your lenses.

63. Never mix solutions from different manufacturers.

64. Do not reuse the remaining solution in your lens case after removing your contact lenses. Discard it and use fresh solution when you are ready for your next cleaning process.

From the bitterness of disease man learns the sweetness of health.

~ Catalan Proverb

65.   Never wet your contact lens with your saliva. The risk of infection is very high.

66.   Your contact lens case can collect all kinds of bacteria, so you should wash it often. Wash your case with soap and rinse it with boiled water.

67.   Replace your contact lens case every three to four months.

68.   Try to change into glasses in the evenings. Most lenses are only designed to be worn for ten to twelve hours.

69.   If you can, try extended-wear lenses: You can wear them safely for a week (or a month), without removing them.

70.   Daily disposable lenses should be replaced daily, two weeks replacement lenses should be replaced every two weeks, and so on. Even though the quality of the lens itself might not decline, protein build-up will make your vision less clear, and there is a higher risk for infections.

The greatest wealth is health.

~ Virgil

71.   Never swap lenses with other people. This is a sure way to pick up an eye infection.

72.   Never wear contact lenses while swimming or using the hot tub.

73.   Never let creams or lotions come in contact with the lenses.

74.   Avoid lash-extending mascara, which has fibers that can irritate the eyes.

75.   Avoid waterproof mascara because it cannot be easily removed with water. It may stain the lenses.

76.   Keep false eyelash adhesive, nail polish and remover, perfume, and cologne away from lenses because they can damage the plastic.

77.   Buy colored lenses from a reputable source. Even if it is part of a costume for party wear (or Halloween) and you may wear it only once, buy it from a reputable source.

A Short History of Medicine
2000 BC "Here, eat this root."
1000 BC "That root is heathen, say this prayer."
AD 1850 "That prayer is superstition, drink this potion."
AD 1940 "That potion is snake oil, swallow this pill."
AD 1985 "That pill is ineffective, take this antibiotic."
AD 2000 "That antibiotic is artificial. Here, eat this root."

~ Author Unknown

78. For colored lenses: Even if you have perfect vision, the actual fit of the lenses must be prescribed.

79. Check the expiration date before using the lenses.

Early to bed and early to rise makes a man healthy, wealthy, and wise.

~ Benjamin Franklin

80. Eyexercise 2

Sit comfortably and take deep breaths.

Move your eyes upward as far as you can.

Then move them downward as far as you can.

Repeat four more times.

Blink a few times. Then, close your eyes and relax for a minute.

> **Symptoms, then, are in reality nothing but the cry from suffering organs.**
>
> **~ Jean Martin Charcot, translated from French**

81. Drink adequate water to prevent dehydration, which usually causes dry eyes.

82. Air conditioning and heating can cause dry eyes. Use a humidifier. Also, avoid sitting very close directly in front of the heater.

83. Too much caffeinated beverages can cause dehydration. Avoid or reduce caffeine. Substitute some of your caffeinated drinks with noncaffeinated beverages.

84. Staring at the computer monitor or TV, and even reading, can cause dry eyes. Take frequent breaks. (See tips in other sections.)

85. Smoking can cause dry eyes. Try to avoid being exposed to second-hand smoke. If your partner, friend, or colleague smokes, firmly set your limits. If it doesn't work, just make sure you're not getting the whole smoke experience without the actual smoking.

86. Taking Omega 3 capsules can help dry eyes. Do consult your physician before doing so.

Water is the only drink for a wise man.

~ Henry David Thoreau

87. Water, water, water: Drink this glorious liquid to keep every cell in your body (including your eyes) lubricated. It helps in preventing dry eyes.

88. We can become dehydrated so gradually that we do not notice the change. For optimum care of eyes, keep yourself hydrated.

89. Caffeine (in coffee, chocolate, soft drinks, etc.) can cause dehydration. Reduce your caffeine intake and drink more decaffeinated liquids.

90. When you drink a cup of coffee or tea, drink a glass of water with it.

Fasting and natural diet, though essentially unknown [in today's U.S.] as a therapy, should be the first treatment when someone discovers that she or he has a medical problem. It should not be applied only to the most advanced cases, as is present practice. Whether the patient has a cardiac condition, hypertension, autoimmune disease, fibroids, or asthma, he or she must be informed that fasting and natural, plant-based diets are a viable alternative to conventional therapy, and an effective one. The time may come when not offering this substantially more effective nutritional approach will be considered malpractice.

~ Joel Fuhrman, M.D.

91. Avoid when you can, or minimize if you must, contact with chemicals—hair spray, perfumes, toner, etc. If your eyes feel discomfort when using a chemical, minimize the use. If your eyes sting or water when you use a chemical product, try to avoid using it.

92. Wherever possible, try to use soap and chemical-free face wash, organic eye creams and makeup, and chemical-free items.

93. Try to use chemical-free cleansers to clean your house. Try a steam cleaner if you can.

Everyone has a doctor in him or her; we just have to help it in its work. The natural healing force within each one of us is the greatest force in getting well.

~ Hippocrates

94.   Once in a while, anybody can get blurry vision, but it is resolved quickly. If it doesn't, or if it happens often, consult your doctor.

95.   Diabetes can also cause blurry vision due to edema. Consult your doctor.

96.   Blurry vision can also be a warning of onset of diabetes. The excess sugar can cause the natural lens to change its shape, causing temporary visual change. Unusual thirst and frequent urination are other symptoms of diabetes. Have yourself tested as soon as possible and keep your blood sugar levels steady.

97.   Diabetes is a big enemy of healthy eyes. Diabetes can affect every part of the eye and can result in refractive error, cataracts, glaucoma diabetic retinopathy, macular degeneration etc. If you're diabetic, take extra good care of your eyes.

Man may be the captain of his fate, but is also the victim of his blood sugar.

~ Wilfrid G. Oakley

98.   Diabetic retinopathy often has no early symptoms. It is vital for all diabetics to have a yearly eye exam.

99.   For those of you who are at high risk, the ideal solution is to avoid diabetes (especially type 2). Staying in shape, not being overweight, regular exercise, and sensible eating habits (I know I've oversimplified the rules!!!) can help you.

100.   It is not always possible to avoid diabetes, especially when hereditary factors are involved. If you're diagnosed with diabetes, try to keep your blood glucose level as close to normal as possible.

101.   Diabetics should eat at regular intervals to prevent the blood sugar from shooting up and down.

To be silent the whole day long, see no newspaper, hear no radio, listen to no gossip, be thoroughly and completely lazy, thoroughly and completely indifferent to the fate of the world is the finest medicine a man can give himself.

~ Henry Miller

102. A healthy, balanced diet with lots of vegetables and fruits and a lesser quantity of animal fats may help prevent cataract formation.

103. Age is the primary risk factor for cataracts. Some of the other factors include diabetes, family history, smoking, alcoholism, obesity, previous eye surgery and excessive exposure to sunlight. Have a thorough eye exam when you turn forty. After that, do get yourself checked every year even if you have no risk factors. But, rest assured that many people with high risk factors do not develop cataracts.

104. Once you are diagnosed with cataract, surgery is the only recourse (as of now).

105. The success rate in cataract surgery is very high. Percentages apart, remember every surgery has its own risks.

106. After the surgery, even though your surgeon may say it's OK to read and watch TV, take it easy. Don't burden your eyes.

> *We are living in a world today where lemonade is made from artificial flavors and furniture polish is made from real lemons.*
>
> *~Alfred E. Newman*

107. After cataract surgery, modify your diet. Reduce sugar, reduce salt, and increase fresh vegetables.

108. For some people, the lens capsule may get cloudy after the surgery. This usually happens within a year or two. Fortunately, this can be easily solved with a special laser treatment.

Our life is frittered away by detail. An honest man has hardly need to count more than his ten fingers, or in extreme cases he may add his ten toes, and lump the rest. Simplicity, simplicity, simplicity!

~ Henry David Thoreau

109. Glaucoma has no cure (as of now). If you're diagnosed with it, use eye drops as prescribed and eat sensibly.

110. Glaucoma can creep up with almost no symptoms. Although anyone can get glaucoma, diabetes, family history, blood pressure, short sightedness, and eye injuries are some of risk factors. Even if you have no risk factors, have yearly eye exams after you turn forty.

I am getting to an age when I can only enjoy the last sport left. It is called hunting for your spectacles.

~ Edward Grey

111. Try to remove these ageing factors from your life. These have a viselike grip, so get professional help if needed. These make you look older and age faster, and bring about many health problems. The appearance of your eyes is a big factor in determining youth and vitality.

> i) Smoking (causes wrinkles in your face, around your eyes, etc.)
> ii) Alcohol (causes puffy eyes)
> iii) Too much salt (causes puffy eyes, swollen eyes, etc.)
> iv) Sleep deprivation (causes puffy eyes, dull eyes, etc.)

There's so much pollution in the air now that if it weren't for our lungs there'd be no place to put it all.

~ Robert Orben

112. We emphasize the havoc pollution causes to our lungs and respiratory organs. We often ignore the fact that pollution taxes and tires our eyes.

113. If you live in or are visiting a polluted city, avoid going out in the middle of the day. The pollution from the heavy traffic and the heat can be dangerous.

114. Use glasses to help eyes navigate the pollution.

115. If you live in a polluted city, have a cool or lukewarm shower or bath when you get home in the evening. Or, wash your face, hands, and feet in cool or lukewarm water.

***Our houses are such unwieldy property that we are
often imprisoned rather than housed in them.***

~ Henry David Thoreau

116. Dust is irritating to the eyes.

117. Try to minimize exposure to dust in your daily life.

118. Use a moistened cloth or tissue to wipe surfaces in your
      home.

119. Try to vacuum and wash your floors as often as necessary.
      If you can draw dust bunnies, then you've waited too
      long.

Dost thou love life? Then do not squander time, for that is the stuff life is made of.

~ Benjamin Franklin

These eye-friendly tips help you save time:

120. Use cucumber slices or teabags when you're planning to take a footbath.

121. Listen to the news on the radio while washing up or dusting. Your muscles get a workout while you get updated on current affairs or sashay to your favorite tunes; all this with minimum eyestrain.

122. Exercise in front of the TV if you can. You see less than half of your serial while getting a workout and reducing eyestrain. At the same time, you're updated as you'll be *hearing* your show.

A pessimist sees the difficulty in every opportunity;
an optimist sees the opportunity in every difficulty.

~ Winston Churchill

I was single when I moved to a new country, which had winters colder than I had imagined. For the first time in my life, I got to know my TV and spent Saturday nights watching movies. That's when I discovered the power of commercial breaks.

I usually sat down with my dinner fifteen or twenty minutes before the movie started. I sat down with my book or magazine or the mail. This way, I was not stressed and was also able to catch up with my reading. And, it gave me time to enjoy my food.

Here is how I spent the commercial breaks.

First break: Dashed to the kitchen with my plate, salsa, etc. Started the kettle. Made herbal tea or a skinny latte. Walked back to the sofa with a yummy hot cup. I enjoyed my tea with the movie.

Second break: Hopped to the kitchen—cleared and cleaned the oven tops. Stacked dishes in the dishwasher. Checked if doors and windows were locked. Danced back to the sofa.

Third break: Called my friend for a chat or sent a text message. Jogged around the house and turned off heaters and other electric appliances. Marched back to the couch.

Fourth break: Dashed to the bathroom: brushed teeth, flossed, washed and dried face and feet. Wafted back to the sofa with face cream and foot cream and socks.

Applied creams. Put on socks. Did these chores after the movie started.

When the movie was over, I turned off the TV and sashayed to the bedroom and turned in.

Most of my colleagues and friends complained about the commercial breaks. In fact, they usually spent it flicking through the channels and getting bored. I got my chores done and got enough breaks from staring at the TV.

Now, no longer single, I've revised my routine, and it includes many chores. Sometimes it doesn't work. Then, I either do some yoga or curl up and read during the breaks.

So, how can this help you if you're a single mum of two?
Use the first break to tuck in your tots and adapt the rest. Once you start planning, you'll get the hang of it and make a success of using the ad breaks wisely and avoid eyestrain.

What if you're married and your wife doesn't share your enthusiasm?
Use one break on her to massage her feet or give her a backrub. Tell her that you're reserving one break for her every time there's a movie with ad breaks. She'll become a fan and will help you adapt the routine.

EMOTION, *n. A prostrating disease caused by a determination of the heart to the head. It is sometimes accompanied by a copious discharge of hydrated chloride of sodium from the eyes.*

~ Ambrose Bierce

123. Blink often. Healthy normal blinking takes place fifteen to twenty times per minute. This can prevent dry eyes.

124. Staring at the computer monitor or TV, or even reading, reduces blinking. This can lead to dry eyes.

125. If your eyes feel dry while you're watching TV or reading, take a break. Close your eyes and then blink slowly a few times.

A custom loathsome to the eye, hateful to the nose, harmful to the brain, dangerous to the lungs, and in the black, stinking fume thereof nearest resembling the horrible Stygian smoke of the pit that is bottomless.

~ *James I of England,* A Counterblaste to Tobacco, *1604*

126. Do you smoke? There are so many health reasons to give up smoking. But let's concentrate on the cosmetic reason: Smoking can give you wrinkles in your face and around your eyes. This ages you faster and you look older. Do you want to look forty-eight when you're thirty-three?

127. Smoking gives you dry eyes.

128. Make sure you don't get exposed to passive smoke. It's of little use that you don't smoke if you're sitting next to a smoker.

Every form of addiction is bad, no matter whether the narcotic be alcohol or morphine or idealism.

~ Carl Jung

129. Alcohol, apart from all the health damages it causes, can make you look older because of puffy eyes.

130. Alcohol can dehydrate you. Drink a glass of water with a glass of alcoholic beverage.

> **The doctor of the future will give no medication, but will interest his patients in the care of the human frame, diet and in the cause and prevention of disease.**
>
> **~ Thomas Edison**

131. Always consult your doctor before you begin to take any medication—even vitamins.

132. If you've been sedentary for a while, consult your doctor before beginning to exercise. Also, do get your doctor's advice before any changes to your exercise routine.

133. Choose your doctor with care if you have the opportunity to do so. Let pep and positive attitude be the deciding factor where experience and talent are similar.

Let food be thy medicine, thy medicine shall be thy food.

~ Hippocrates

134. Vitamins C and E are vital for eye health.

135. Try to drink a glass of orange/lemon/lime juice daily (except if you're allergic to citrus fruits or taking certain medications).

136. Take vitamin C supplements if you're over fifty, have eye conditions, etc.

137. Vitamin C is vital if you're recovering from surgery or illness.

138. Instead of paying extravagantly for vegetable extracts, try to incorporate these vegetables in your diet. Green beans, broccoli, Brussel sprouts, tomatoes, carrots, spinach, celery, leeks, lettuce, peas, squash, and turnips: All these get gold medals for eye health. Include them often in your diet.

139. Eat carrots at least four to five times a week. Carrots have beta carotene, the precursor to Vitamin A. Even if you pay a lot to buy antiaging creams with retinol (Vitamin A), try to include carrots, preferably raw, in your diet. If you're diabetic, do not eat boiled carrots and limit yourself to one medium-sized raw carrot per day.

When diet is wrong medicine is of no use.
When diet is correct medicine is of no need.

~ *Ayurvedic Proverb*

140. Zinc is vital for eye health. It may help delay age-related macular degeneration. Make sure your diet contains sunflower seeds, pumpkin seeds, beans, wheat germ, almonds, nuts, etc. Oysters and red meat are excellent sources of zinc. If you're a vegetarian or vegan, take a zinc supplement once or twice a week.

141. Lycopene is supposed to promote eye health. Tomatoes are a rich source of lycopene. Best when the tomatoes are cooked and with some oil. Try to include pasta sauce one to two times a week.

142. Lutein is supposed to promote eye health. Fruit, berries, and vegetables with red, orange, and yellow pigments— such as carrots, squash, and tomatoes—are sources of lutein. Vegetables rich in beta carotene are also rich in lutein.

143. Take lutein supplements if you have vision problems.

144. Try to eat spinach at least once a week. Add it to your soup or salad or your main dish.

Walking: the most ancient exercise and still the best modern exercise.

~ Carrie Latet

145. Eyexercise 3

Sit comfortably and take deep breaths.

Move your eyes to your right and left at eye level.

Keep your raised fingers on each side as guides and adjust them so that you can see them clearly when moving the eyes to the right and to the left, but without straining.

Keeping the fingers at eye level, and moving only the eyes, look to the right at your chosen point, then to the left.

Repeat three times.

Blink a few times, and then close your eyes and rest.

*All human situations have their own inconveniences.
We feel those of the present but neither see nor
feel those of the future; and hence we often make
troublesome changes without amendment, and
frequently for the worse.*

~ Benjamin Franklin

146. If you're pregnant, you need to care extra for your eyes. It's very easy to neglect one's eyes during pregnancy.

147. If you're pregnant and you wear glasses, have an eye exam because pregnancy may require a change of prescription.

148. Minimize the use of contact lenses during pregnancy.

149. Regular low-impact exercise is very important for a healthy pregnancy to prevent gestational diabetes. Diabetes is the enemy of healthy eyes.

There is one thing more exasperating than a wife who can cook and won't, and that's a wife who can't cook and will.

~ Robert Frost

150. *Eye-deal snack*

This is my own recipe for a quick and tasty snack, good for your eyes. There are many different ways to adapt it to suit your taste, time, and needs. Let your imagination fly with your taste buds. You can substitute nuts, seeds, and veggies according to your taste.

Buy organic carrots if you can. Wash, peel, and grate carrots. Peel only a very thin layer. Store the grated carrots in your fridge. Use them within three to four days.

Open a can of brown beans and rinse thoroughly. Keep them in a glass container in the fridge and use within three to four days.

o   Take a bowlful of grated carrots when you feel like snacking.

o   Chop some vegetables and herbs according to your taste: celery, capsicum, onion, cucumber, fennel, tomato, etc. Add them to the grated carrot. Add some nuts of your choice, a few drops of lime juice for the tang, and a spoonful of olive oil or balsamic vinegar dressing. A great salad in five minutes.

o   Diabetic? Add one tomato, a third of a cucumber, and a couple of celery sticks for every three spoons of grated carrots. Garnish with walnuts. Add lime juice instead of dressing.

o Olive fan? Rinse a few olives. This washes off some of the salt. Chop them and add to the carrots. Sprinkle sunflower seeds.

He that eats till he is sick must fast till he is well.

~ English Proverb

o   Indigestion? Add chopped fennel to the grated carrots. Add lime juice. Garnish with mint leaves if you can.

o   You just have a minute? Add a couple of cherry tomatoes, a handful of canned brown beans, and a pinch of pumpkin seeds to the grated carrot: Your salad is ready to go.

o   Want a sweet and healthy snack? Add a few chopped cashew nuts and dried apricots.

o   One-minute sweet salad? Add a few raisins, sunflower seeds, and walnuts to the grated carrots. You have a healthy, sweet snack within half a minute.

A wise man should consider that health is the greatest of human blessings, and learn how by his own thought to derive benefit from his illnesses.

~ Hippocrates

151. Wash your hands before using eye drops or ointment.

152. Be careful not to let the tip of the dropper touch any part of your eye.

153. While tilting your head back, pull the lower eyelid down with one or two fingers to create a small pouch. Gently squeeze the dropper to put the eye drops or a thin line of ointment in the pouch. Close the eye for thirty to sixty seconds to let the drops move around.

154. If shaky hands are a problem while using eye drops, try using a wrist weight (one pound, or half a kilo). These are usually available from sporting good stores. The extra weight can decrease mild shaking.

155. Store the eye drops or ointment properly. Read the instructions.

156. Do not use more drops or ointment than directed.

157. When you open the vial or tube, write the date on its label. Toss it out after the recommended period even if it is not used up.

Our own physical body possesses a wisdom which we who inhabit the body lack. We give it orders which make no sense.

~ Henry Miller

158. Most eye infections can be avoided by basic hygiene rules.

159. Wash hands after visiting the toilet.

160. After touching or playing with pets, wash your hands.

161. As part of your routine when you return home (even after a quick trip to the neighbor), wash your hands first.

162. Have a liquid disinfectant (the type that requires no water) in your bag, car, desk, etc. It is useful when you're away from soap and water.

163. Wipe all surfaces, door handles, switches, garbage can covers, telephones, mailbox, etc., with very dilute chlorine. Do it every six weeks. If you use an environmentally friendly solution, do it every three to four weeks.

Leave your drugs in the chemist's post if you can heal the patient with food.

~ Hippocrates

164. Too much salt in the diet can affect many organs, including eyes.

165. A low-salt diet can prevent cosmetic problems such as puffy eyes. Puffy eyes make you look older.

166. A low-salt diet can also prevent serious conditions such as cataracts.

167. If you use more herbs, you can gradually reduce the salt in your diet.

Every man is the builder of a temple called his body.

~ Henry David Thoreau

168. Sugar is a big enemy of healthy eyes. It should be used sparingly even if you're not a diabetic.

169. It's very unhealthy for eyes to let your blood sugar shoot up and down (even if you're not a diabetic).

Life well spent is long.

~ *Leonardo da Vinci*

The glycemic index (GI) is a numerical system of measuring how much of a rise in circulating blood sugar a carbohydrate triggers—the higher the number, the greater the blood sugar response. So a low GI food will cause a small rise, while a high GI food will trigger a dramatic spike. A GI of 70 or more is high, a GI of 56 to 69 is medium, and a GI of 55 or less is low.

The glycemic load (GL) is a relatively new way to assess the impact of carbohydrate consumption that takes the glycemic index into account, but gives a fuller picture than does glycemic index alone. A GL of 20 or more is high, a GL of 11 to 19 inclusive is medium, and a GL of 10 or less is low. A GI value tells you only how rapidly a particular carbohydrate turns into sugar. It doesn't tell you how much of that carbohydrate is in a serving of a particular food. You need to know both things to understand a food's effect on blood sugar. That is where glycemic load comes in. The carbohydrate in watermelon, for example, has a high GI. But there isn't a lot of it, so watermelon's glycemic load is relatively low.

(www.officialdiabetesblog.com)

One of the first duties of the physician is to educate the masses not to take medicine.

~ Sir William Osler

170. If you're a diabetic or have any eye condition, acquaint yourself with GI/GL of foods. Consult a nutritional consultant if you can.

171. Avoid white bread, white rice, sugary snacks, and sweet desserts. This is not just for diabetics, but for anyone who wants to take care of their eyes for old age.

172. Limit starchy or root vegetables and fruits like bananas, jackfruits, and melons. Avoid these if you're a diabetic.

173. Try to eat low GI and GL foods. This helps in maintaining a stable blood glucose level and should be the first step toward maintaining healthy eyes.

174. *Here's a quick basic summary, which is definitely incomplete, for starters:*

> i) Citrus fruits have lower GI than starchy fruits (bananas, for example).

> ii) Starchy (and root) vegetables have higher GI than leafy vegetables.

> iii) Unrefined and less processed grains have lower GI. Grains have lower GI than flour.

iv) The higher the fiber and the lower the processing, the lower the GI (usually).

An ounce of prevention is worth a pound of cure.

~ Benjamin Franklin

175. During their season, try to substitute berries for snacks.

176. If you live in areas where you can buy fresh blueberries during season, try to include them in your diet three to four days a week.

177. Bilberry, blueberry's cousin, has more nutrient value. Eat it whenever you can. Scandinavia, which has bilberry growing wild and cultivated, has named it *blåbær*, blueberry.

178. Don't smother the blueberries with sugar. Sprinkle very little brown sugar or honey on the top. Enjoy the sweet and tangy taste of the berries. Remember, they are loaded with antioxidants, which are good for your eyes.

179. Freeze the fresh berries and use them during winter.

180. If you cannot get blueberries where you live, try to get extracts. Use the minimum dose recommended. (Discuss this with your doctor first.)

Simplicity is the ultimate sophistication.

~ Leonardo da Vinci

181. Stress can cause circles or bags under the eyes, skin disruptions, wrinkles around the eyes, and premature ageing.

182. Try to keep your shoulders low, especially when you're stressed.

183. Roll your head from side to side or in a circular motion. Do it smoothly for a minute.

184. Shrug slowly. Lift your shoulders and sink them gently. Do it a couple of times.

185. Close your eyes for a few seconds and take a few deep breaths.

186. Surround yourself in soothing colors (ocean blue, green pastures, yellow). Let your walls soothe you.

187. Yoga is a gentle stress reliever.

> **All our talents increase in the using, and every faculty, both good and bad, strengthens by exercise.**
>
> *~ Anne Brontë*

188. Eyexercise 4

Sit comfortably.

Look at your chosen point in right corner up, then to the one in left corner down.

Repeat three times.

Blink several times. Close your eyes and rest.

Now do it in reverse. First look to the left corner up, then to the right corner down.

Repeat three times.

Blink several times. Close your eyes and rest.

He who has health has hope, and he who has hope has everything.

~ *Arabic Proverb*

conjunctivitis: inflammation of the conjunctiva (informal name: pink eye)

conjunctiva: the mucus membrane that lines the inner surface of the eyelids and is continued over the forepart of the eyeball.
   (*Merriam-Webster's Medical Desk Dictionary*)

189.   Prevention is the best method to avoid conjunctivitis (pink eye).

190.   Never touch your eyes without washing your hands.

191.   If you do get pink eye, throw out your eye creams and eye makeup.

192.   Use disposable tissues or handkerchiefs during the disease to prevent spreading the infection.

193.   Use a clean tissue to remove discharge from eyes, and wash hands to prevent the spread of infection.

From the bitterness of disease man learns the sweetness of health.

~ Catalan Proverb

sty: an inflamed swelling of the sebaceous gland at the margin of an eyelid
  (*Merriam-Webster's Medical Desk Dictionary*)

194. A sty can be treated by applying a warm, clean, moist cloth to the affected eye for a few minutes, three to four times a day.

195. The abscess should not be squeezed, as this will spread the infection.

196. If the sty fails to go away after a couple of days, contact your doctor.

If I'd known I was going to live so long, I'd have taken better care of myself.

~ Leon Eldred

197. Causes of watery eyes: allergies, infection, or a small foreign body lodged in the eye.

198. Strange but true: Watery eyes can also be a symptom of dry eyes.

199. Seek medical attention if you have prolonged unexplainable excessively watering eyes, painful watery eyes or watery eyes with other symptoms such as sinus pain, etc.

A good laugh and a long sleep are the best cures in the doctor's book.

~ Irish Proverb

200. A jarring blow to the head can cause hemorrhage, or blood in the white of the eye.

201. Hemorrhage can also result from anything that puts too much pressure on these fragile blood vessels, such as uncontrolled blood pressure, childbirth, weight lifting, intense coughing, vomiting, or even sneezing.

202. Seek immediate medical attention if it is accompanied by pain or impaired vision.

203. The blood will slowly be absorbed, and the eye will heal itself within a week or two. Otherwise, consult your doctor.

Do not lose hold of your dreams or aspirations.
For if you do, you may still exist but you have ceased
to live.

~ Henry David Thoreau

204. Flaking eyelids frequently occur in people who have oily skin, dandruff, or dry eyes. Many medications are available for treatment but are not sufficient without the daily cleansing routine.

205. A warm cloth placed over closed eyelids for a few minutes will help to soften crusts and loosen oily debris.

206. Use a prepared eyelid cleansing solution with a cotton ball, cotton swab, or clean cloth to gently scrub the lids for a couple of minutes. Thoroughly rinse the eyelids and pat dry.

I shut my eyes and all the world drops dead;
I lift my eyes and all is born again.

~ Sylvia Plath

207. Twitching of the eyes can be caused by many factors: It can be environmental, physiological, or psychological—lack of sleep, fatigue, epilepsy, stress, anxiety, too much eye stress (too much TV or computer), overconsumption of caffeine, etc.

208. If twitching is accompanied by fever, red eyes, decrease in vision, blurry vision, or pain, consult your doctor at once.

209. If you don't have any other symptoms except the eye twitch, contact your doctor if it increases or doesn't disappear within a day.

To lengthen thy lives, lessen thy meals.

~ Benjamin Franklin

Here's one of my favorite light dinners. This can be adapted to suit many tastes. Let your imagination fly.

o   Soak raisins in cold water overnight. Drain, rinse, and put them away in the fridge. (I usually have a small cup in the fridge at all times as an emergency snack.) Wash, peel (a very thin layer), and grate carrots. Hope you go organic.

o   Take a big bowl. Add two cups of grated carrots and half a cup of raisins. Add a handful of walnuts. Sprinkle a few pine nuts or sunflower seeds. Mix it well with a few drops of lime juice for that tang.

o   Toast two slices of whole grain bread. Spread unsalted butter or peanut butter on one. Spread blueberry jam (or any other fruit jam) on the other. Try to buy peanut butter and jams with no added sugar.

o   Heat skimmed milk. Make decaffeinated instant coffee or steam the milk to make skinny latte or cappuccino.

Enjoy!

o   Substitute peanut butter with lean meat for variety.

o   If you're a vegetarian, substitute one slice with cottage cheese.

o   If you're a vegan, add hummus.

o   If you're diabetic, add half a cup of grated carrots, one cup of chopped celery, and a handful of walnuts. And substitute one rye cake (or Ryvita) for one slice.

o   If you want to reduce your carbohydrates intake, cut out the bread. Have a grilled chicken or poached fish instead.

Bon appétit.

Drugs are not always necessary. Belief in recovery always is.

~ Norman Cousins

210. No child is too young for a complete eye exam.

211. If your baby is premature, make sure the hospital or birthing center thoroughly checks his eyes before you go home. If not, make an appointment to see your eye doctor.

212. When the baby is six months old, the pediatrician should check the baby's eye alignment and visual fixation (how he or she focuses his or her gaze).

213. Doctors have special tests for infants and toddlers that help them to diagnose conditions that are generally invisible to the naked eye. Treating these conditions early decreases the chances that they will develop into more serious or even permanent problems.

214. Children should have a thorough eye exam before age three. Crossed eyes, lazy eye, drooping of the upper eyelid, vision, etc should be checked.

215. Teach your children not to rub their eyes or eyelids on waking up. This could be one of the best youthful gifts you give them.

216. If lazy eye is detected in early childhood, it is treatable.

Life expectancy would grow by leaps and bounds if green vegetables smelled as good as bacon.

~ Doug Larson

217. The earlier the treatment is started for crossed eyes, the better the chance of restoring normal sight. Left untreated, the child could develop permanent visual problems, including lazy eye.

218. When your child starts school, she usually gets an eye exam. If the school does not have one, make sure your child gets a thorough eye exam before beginning school.

219. If your child tilts her head to read, squints or blinks a lot, omits words while reading, rubs her eyes often, has problems throwing or catching objects, contact your doctor. Make sure your child gets a complete eye exam.

220. If your teenagers are using contact lenses, make sure they wear protective goggles for sports.

221. Keep an updated medical journal—this could help your children and grandchildren.

222. Talk to your children and grandchildren about any eye conditions that you have. Get them to look after their eyes from an early age.

Leave all the afternoon for exercise and recreation, which are as necessary as reading. I will rather say more necessary because health is worth more than learning.

~ Thomas Jefferson

223. Don't strain your eyes reading in dim light.

224. If the light is too bright, it can strain your eyes.

225. Never lie flat on your back and read.

226. If you read in bed, place a pillow to support your back and a pillow on your lap.

227. Don't read a book with tiny print if you get a headache within a few minutes of starting to read.

228. While reading, close your eyes after each chapter and take deep breaths.

229. Take a break every half hour while reading. Get up, walk for a couple of minutes, and stretch.

Be careful about reading health books. You may die of a misprint.

~ *Mark Twain*

230. Reading for an hour or more can dry your eyes, as you involuntarily blink at a slower rate. As you turn a page, blink a couple of times.

231. Have adequate light for reading. This depends on age also—a sixty-year-old usually needs more light than a twenty-year-old.

232. Avoid reading in a moving vehicle. Apart from motion sickness, it tires your eyes.

233. The ideal reading distance (somewhere between twelve to twenty inches or thirty to fifty centimetres) may vary from person to person. You don't have to walk around with a scale measuring the distance. But, make sure that you don't strain or squint while reading.

"The wireless music box has no imaginable commercial value. Who would pay for a message sent to nobody in particular?"

~ David Sarnoff's associates in response to his urging for investment in the radio in the 1920s

234. Increase the audio and reduce the video in your daily life to avoid eyestrain.

235. Include the radio in your life. Listen to the news or dance to the music. Just close your eyes and let your ears do the work.

236. Invest in a good audio stereo system. And also begin to use it often.

237. Try to make friends with radio's cousins: cassette player, walkman, CD player, MP3 player, etc. All these allow you to do something else while listening to them.

238. Get a few books on tape, that you might read (listen to) again and again. Enjoy it with your eyes closed or enjoy it with the eye-deal snack.

239. This is a wonderful habit to inculcate in young children: Choose a favorite CD—this is now your special CD— and dance to it. Do it often. Use another CD as a bedtime cue. This beats the *glued to the TV set* syndrome.

[Sleep is] the golden chain that ties health and our bodies together.

~ Thomas Dekker

240. Beauty sleep is not just for the beauties. Restful slumber is vital for eye health.

241. Average sleep required is six to nine hours depending on age, sex, health, habits, routines, etc. Women may require more sleep. As we grow older, our need for sleep decreases. Conditions like low blood pressure and anemia can increase the need for sleep. A fifty-year-old man usually needs less sleep than a thirty-year-old lady. But, if he is an athlete, he might need more sleep. If you do not awake refreshed or need an alarm to wake up, you may not be getting enough sleep. Try to give your body its healing hours.

242. Too little or too much sleep can cause puffy eyes.

243. Get up at a fixed time every day—Sundays and holidays too.

244. Have a bedtime, but be flexible. Give a leeway of an hour either way. Go to bed when you feel sleepy.

245. If you're not sleepy even an hour after your bedtime, just go to bed and close your eyes. Don't panic. Even just closing your eyes in the dark and relaxing is good for your eye health. You may drift into sleep if you don't panic.

Only mad dogs and Englishmen go out in the midday sun.

~ Noel Coward

Siesta—the glorious midday rest or nap. I grew up in south India, where none of the languages have a special word for siesta—we called it afternoon nap or a short nap—but it is practiced by many wise people. In Pondicherry, the former French colony, the shops used to close at noon and open again for business at four in the evening. The French settlers were wise to inculcate the *sieste* routine there.

My mother set a great example for me. She used to take a siesta after lunch. Every day that she was at home, she used to lie down for an hour. OK—her siesta was longer than the Churchill powernap. When we were on a holiday or visiting relatives, it was reduced to fifteen or twenty minutes. She had to lie down after lunch. I used to tease her. I was not a siesta fan. Her standard reply was, "The sun is at its peak. It is a message for us to relax. Laugh all you want to. It's nature's way of telling us to close our eyes and relax for a few minutes."

It was not just the siesta. She avoided going out between noon and two. And she always carried a parasol to protect her hair, face, and neck.

I still remember her baby-soft skin when she was fifty. She had better skin tone than anyone else I knew. Wrinkles around her eyes? You must be joking.

I remember pouting and rubbing my hands on my mom's arms and face. Her skin was soft and silky.

"I want your skin tone. Mom, it's unfair. You have better skin than your own daughter."

"Take care of what you've got," was her standard reply.

I think you might dispense with half your doctors if you would only consult Dr. Sun more.

~ Henry Ward Beecher

246. Sun—a cruel enemy to youth and good looks. Always wear sunglasses and a cap or hat to delay ageing.

247. Sun block—use it if you're going to be in the sun for more than half an hour. Let it be a part of your makeup or routine.

248. Sunbathing may give you a sexy tan. In addition to melanoma and wrinkles, it can also cause cataracts. Use sun block, sunglasses, and a hat. Do not sunbathe every day. Do it occasionally.

249. Never look directly at the sun.

250. If you're hot and tired after a long day in the sun, take a lukewarm or cool shower. Apply moisturizer (or after sun lotion) liberally. Then, close your eyes and place cucumber slices on your eyes for a few minutes. Cucumber is nature's own cooling and soothing agent.

251. Count yourself lucky if you live in the tropics or an area that receives sunshine most of the year. But it is vital both for health and cosmetic reasons not to leave home without sunglasses and a cap or visor.

Water, air, and cleanliness are the chief articles in my pharmacopoeia.

~ Napoleon I

252. If possible, wear close-fitting, wraparound sunglasses. It's worth taking the time to choose a good fitting pair.

253. Check that your sunglasses have adequate UV protection.

254. Myth: The darker the glasses, the better the protection. Sorry. The darkness of the glasses has nothing to do with UV protection.

255. Price does not determine the quality or UV protection of the glasses.

256. Wear sunglasses even on windy days. You protect your eyes from debris flying around.

257. Wearing sunglasses can prevent cataracts (thickening of the lens).

To eat is a necessity, but to eat intelligently is an art.

~ La Rochefoucauld

258. Quiz: ***Amazing, but true***

Q: Gram for gram, what contains more than double the calcium in milk, vitamin C in oranges, protein in yogurt, vitamin A in carrots, and potassium in bananas?

It is eye's best friend.
A: Moringa Oleifera

Tell me what you eat, and I will tell you what you are.

~ Anthelme Brillat-Savarin

Moringa Oleifera—drumstick tree. The fruits resemble drumsticks. Its origin is in the south Indian state of Tamil Nadu (the state where I grew up). It's used in Ayurveda. An old saying claims that it can prevent three hundred diseases. The claim might, or might not be true. But it is your ally for eye health. It is an herbal multivitamin that does wonders for your eyes.

I don't think the scientific *proof* is there yet, but I've seen the benefits while growing up. Our eyes get the maximum benefit from the leaves. It's unfortunate that most people don't like the strong taste of the leaves and just use the yummy drumsticks. Almost everyone in that state ate drumsticks, but few used the leaves.

Growing up in Neyveli, a town in Tamil Nadu, we had a huge drumstick tree in our garden. It must have been four to five meters (twelve to fifteen feet) high. It was huge. We relished the fruits, but the leaves were eaten once every few months only. One day our gardener sobbed that his brother's night vision was reduced. He was a truck driver and might even lose his job. He had three small children and his wife was pregnant. My mom consoled our gardener and told him she would help his brother. When they turned up the next day, she advised him to eat the drumstick leaves. She told them to help themselves to moringa leaves from our tree. She also advised his pregnant wife to eat the leaves. Within a few weeks, he was able to notice that his night vision improved. I was ten or eleven at that time, but I still remember the hoopla when he came with his family to thank my mom. I thought my mom had performed a miracle.

I was convinced that the moringa was a miracle food when I saw many people reverse minor problems of the eye, especially the starting stage of night blindness, by beginning to eat moringa. My mom was a firm believer in its use for night blindness, and we saw many more miracles. She also advised them to see the eye doctor and check things out even though they seemed cured, and to eat moringa leaves at least once every fortnight. Throughout my childhood and adolescence, I remember people coming over to pluck the leaves from our moringa tree. That tree flourished, and when I went to university, it was still swaying proudly.

My mom helped quite a few people who lived below the poverty line. She thought their diet was inadequate and lacking in the correct vitamins. She was sorry for them, as they usually couldn't afford vitamin pills. She wasn't sure if moringa leaves were better than vitamin pills, but they worked wonders. Again, she did not know what they contained, but it was proved over and over that they were vital for eye health.

If you're lucky to live in a place where you can have moringa in your backyard, do use the leaves and not just the yummy drumsticks. If you live in a place where you can buy the leaves, use them regularly. I saw it in an Indian (or maybe Sri Lankan) shop in the United States. I've seen it in a Sri Lankan shop in London. I know that this is available in Southeast Asia. Use this herbal multivitamin for your eyes.

> *Our body is a machine for living. It is organized for that, it is its nature. Let life go on in it unhindered and let it defend itself, it will do more than if you paralyze it by encumbering it with remedies.*
>
> *~ Leo Tolstoy*

259. You cannot be too careful when it comes to sharp pointed objects. Keys, pencils, forks, etc. are used on a daily basis, and we forget that they can be dangerous if we are not careful.

260. Wear safety goggles when required. They might not be sexy, but don't gamble with the safety of your eyes.

261. Firecrackers may give you a thrill, but use goggles to avoid any unpleasant accidents.

262. One of the best gifts to your children is to inculcate in them a sense of safety from their tender ages. It is great to be adventurous, but also follow the safety guidelines.

EMERGENCIES

I am not a health professional, so these are recommendations only. The basic rule is: Your eyes are your most precious possessions. Try to be careful and not take any unnecessary risks. If anything drastic occurs, dial emergency at once.

263. What's the number for 911? Its 112 in most EU and some European countries. In some countries it is a local number. Whether you move to a new city or travelling around, acquaint yourself with the emergency number to call, emergency services, locations, maps, etc. Be prepared for any emergency, even though it may never happen. Get the information before you arrive.

264. In addition, if you move to a new country, you ought to learn a few basic words in the local language. "Fire," "pain," "help," "yes," "no," "left," "right," etc.—these might be invaluable in an emergency.

265. For acid and chemical burns, dial emergency at once. Flush with water at once. Repeat every few minutes till the chemical is out.

266. Abrupt loss of vision, even if painless, is an acute emergency and has to be treated at once.

267. Objects piercing or entering the eyes is an extreme emergency. Do not rub the eye or pull out any object (even a contact lens) from the eye. If you're far from medical attention, cover the eye with a bandage, eye

shield, or a paper cup and tape it while you wait for the ambulance.

268. If cleaning liquids or soaps enter your eye, flush the eye with water. You may have to wash the eyes at least five to ten minutes to get rid of the chemicals.

Health is worth more than learning.

~ Thomas Jefferson

269. Snow blindness is a painful condition that is caused by exposure to sunlight reflected from large expanses of snow or ice. Prevent this by using sunglasses or goggles. If afflicted, seek medical help.

270. Cool air can cause dry eyes. It also dries the mucus membrane of the nose. Drinking water and keeping hydrated helps.

271. It is better to use glasses instead of contact lenses while spending time outdoors.

272. Dry eyes can also be a problem indoors due to heating. Try a humidifier and keep hydrated.

Children are like wet cement. Whatever falls on them makes an impression.

~ Dr. Haim Ginott

273. Teach your children good eye habits from an early age.

274. Toys—from crayons to toy guns—are a major source of injury, so check all toys for sharp or pointed parts.

275. Teach children that any kind of missile, projectile, or BB gun is not a toy.

276. Be a good role model—always wear proper eye protection.

277. Get protective eyewear for your children and help them use it properly.

278. Teach children that flying toys should never be pointed at another person.

A wise man should consider that health is the greatest
of human blessings, and learn how by his own thought
to derive benefit from his illnesses.

~ Hippocrates

279. Teach children how to carry sharp or pointed objects properly.

280. Discourage the purchase and use of firecrackers in the home.

281. Don't let children or teenagers light explosive firecrackers.

282. Use safety measures near fires and explosives, such as campfires and fireworks.

283. If you swim, use goggles. It is not a beauty aid, but your eyes will thank you.

284. Wear polarized sunglasses if you're an outdoor sportsperson.

285. Use the specific safety equipment appropriate for the sport: helmet, goggles, etc.

> **To be seventy years young is sometimes far more cheerful and hopeful than to be forty years old.**
>
> *~ Oliver Wendell Holmes*

286. If you're over fifty and have a habit of reading the newspaper every morning, try to incorporate the radio into your life. Listen to the news while sipping your juice or herbal tea. It's not the same, but your eyes will thank you.

287. As you grow older—preferably by age fifty-five to sixty—change the lights in your home. Get brighter lights.

288. Make sure you have adequate light for reading.

289. Buy a good magnifying glass if you are troubled by small print. Buy a magnifying page if you're going to use it to read a book. Use these aids to avoid unnecessary strain.

290. Carry a magnifying glass with you. You can avoid squinting when you're on the move.

291. Get an enlarged telephone dial to avoid the extra strain.

292. Buy a calculator with oversized numbers and a big display to minimize strain.

293. Try to buy books that you use often in large print—dictionary, thesaurus, etc. At least, don't get the tiniest print in the market.

***The art of medicine consists in amusing the patient
while nature cures the disease.***

~ Voltaire

294. Balance your hobbies—if one of your hobbies causes a
      lot of eyestrain, include activities that are easy on your
      eyes. If reading is your hobby, try to include some radio
      instead of TV.

295. If sewing is one of your hobbies, make sure you adjust
      your posture and light so that your eyes don't suffer as
      you grow older.

To avoid sickness eat less; to prolong life worry less.

~ Chu Hui Weng

296. Don't flock to "see" a beautiful solar eclipse. You should never look directly at the sun (eclipse or otherwise).

297. If you really want to watch an eclipse, do so with special goggles.

298. When your friends and family are getting busy with glasses to watch an eclipse, relax. Enjoy the time in. Watch a DVD with your kids or spend some time with your parents.

Mother Nature gave us eyelids. She didn't give us earlids or bodylids.

~ Steven Halpern

299. *Eyexercise 5 (Massage)*

Close your eyes and lightly and gently stroke the lids with your fingertips.

Back and forth, top and bottom, lids as well.

Don't do it unless your fingernails are trimmed short.

After these two, Dr. Diet and Dr. Quiet, Dr. Merriman is requisite to preserve health.

~ *James Howell*

Puffy eyes

The following can cause puffy eyes:

(a) Alcohol
(b) Too little or too much sleep
(c) Too much salt in the diet

Solution:

Teabags on the eyes

To get rid of bags under your eyes, you can place used tea bags over your eyes. Rinse the bags well in cold water and wring them so that they do not drip. Place the bags over your eyes; leave them for a few minutes. Watch your eyes sparkle.

Life is not merely to be alive, but to be well.

~ Marcus Valerius Martial

300. Slice one small piece off of a potato, and cut the slice in half. Put each slice under your eyes and leave them under your eyes for a few minutes. This reduces dark circles.

301. Freeze some grated cucumbers in an ice tray. Massage frozen cucumber cubes onto eyes to reduce puffiness and dark circles.

Health is my expected heaven.

~ John Keats

Summer day?

Cut two cucumber slices. (Use the rest in your salad). Settle yourself comfortably and play your favorite CD. Close your eyes and place the cucumber slices on your eyes for five minutes. Remove the slices and splash some cool water on your face. Watch your eyes sparkle.

If you have children, let them watch their favorite DVD. Or, make it a family break.

Spouses can do this together. Hold hands while listening to your music.

Anyone who believes that anything can be suited to everyone is a great fool, because medicine is practised not on mankind in general, but on every individual in particular.

~ Henri de Mondeville

302. For black eyes, forget the steak. Take a package of frozen peas and wrap it in a thin cloth. Or take a cold, wet cloth. Leave it on the bruised area for a few minutes, and then take it off for a couple of minutes. Repeat a couple of times.

Eat ripe pineapple and ripe papaya—lots of it—for two or three days, and let the enzymes in those fruits help eliminate the discoloration around the eye.

If you suffer from dryness in addition to discolored circles, use cotton wool soaked in cold milk. Leave it on for a few minutes. Rinse your face clean with lukewarm water.

What fools indeed we mortals are
To lavish care upon a Car,
With ne'er a bit of time to see
About our own machinery!

~ *John Kendrick Bangs*

303. To soothe your tired eyes, place cucumber slices or teabags. Or, squeeze cotton pads out of ice water, place on eyelids, and lie down; elevate your feet.

DONATING THE GIFT OF SIGHT

This is my personal opinion. Do it if you want to. But please read about it if you're not sure. Contact an agency in your area that does this and ask for information.

After you've passed on, your organs are not of use to you. Let two people get the gift of sight after you. Have a donor card in your wallet or handbag. Talk to your spouse, children, doctor, and friends about it.

Almost anyone of any age can pledge to donate their eyes after death. Usually only the cornea (the clear, transparent tissue in front of the eye) is transplanted. It does not matter even if you wear glasses, are hypertensive, are diabetic, or have undergone any eye surgery.

While cornea transplants make up the majority of eye transplant procedures, the sclera (or "white" of the eye) can also be transplanted.

Great care is taken to preserve the appearance of the donor. After donation, it is possible to have an open-casket funeral.